STOP
GAINING
WEIGHT

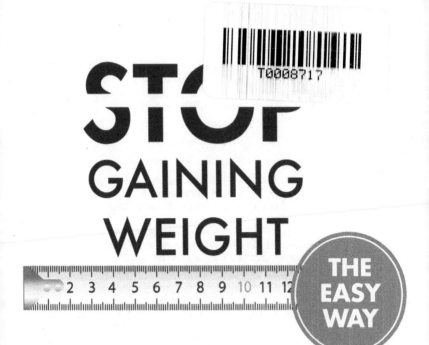

THE EASY WAY

How to maintain a healthy body and mind

**DR MIKE DILKES &
ALEXANDER ADAMS**

First published in Great Britain in 2022 by Orion Spring
an imprint of The Orion Publishing Group Ltd
Carmelite House, 50 Victoria Embankment
London EC4Y 0DZ

An Hachette UK Company

1 3 5 7 9 10 8 6 4 2

A CIP catalogue record for this book is
available from the British Library.

ISBN (Mass Market Paperback) 978 1 8418 8279 6
ISBN (eBook) 978 1 8418 8280 2

Printed and bound in Great Britain by
Clays Ltd, Elcograf, S.p.A

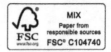

www.orionbooks.co.uk

ORION
SPRING

Contents

Introduction

In 2016 and 2017 the top five searches in Google – aside from those relating to Donald Trump, the Olympic Games and Brexit – related to calories. More specifically, hundreds of millions of searches asking 'How many calories are in … a Big Mac/Quinoa/Wine/ Eggplant?' In 2018, alongside searches for 'What is Bitcoin?', we mainly enquired as to the 'most effective diets?' with the Keto, the Dubrow, Noom and Mediterranean diets all taking the lion's share of the captive audience.

You might be thinking, so what? The world has been obsessed with cellulite, quick-fix diets, celebrity slimming secrets, bum lifts and dad bods for decades. And you would be right. Weight loss and gain has long been a mainstay of the public lexicon; indeed, it may surprise you to learn that colonic irrigation dates back 3000 years to the Egyptians and that Jesus himself refers to it in the 'Essence Gospel of Peace' (allegedly).[1]

There has never been more information and actionable advice about weight loss in human history. A back catalogue which is growing at a pace on a daily basis. And yet we are, by some margin, the fattest global population on record. Worldwide obesity has nearly tripled since 1975 and today 1.9 billion adults are overweight.[2] In the UK alone, at the time of writing, an astonishing 67 per cent of adult men and 60 per cent of adult women are overweight. An example now firmly set for our children, with 20 per cent of 10- to 11-year-olds also officially obese.[3]

Many have a 'live by the sword, die by the sword' attitude to their own weight gain, making clear that their body is their own private kingdom and they are entitled to use it and abuse it as they see fit. Indeed, the wisdom of a viral internet meme tells us that 'couples who truly love each other gain weight together'. Unfortunately, views such as these are at best misguided and at worst inexcusably ignorant, particularly when we consider the societal cost of being overweight. Currently, the UK annual spend on obesity and diabetes stands at £6.9 billion pounds. To put this is into perspective, this is more than is spent each year on the police, the fire service and judicial system ... combined![4]

Perhaps it would more logically follow that couples who truly love each other die of completely preventable illnesses together? (But we suspect the amount of traction this would get versus its predecessor is debatable.)

It is staggering therefore to think that in the age of abundant information, weight-centric cookery shows and a relentless social focus on body aesthetics, obesity would be an issue at all. And yet our problematic waistlines show no sign of abating, with predictions from the medical industry warning of far worsening states of affairs.

Immediately following the Covid-19 outbreak, physicians, family doctors and GPs reported a significant increase in patients' weight.[5] These unexpected pounds are the result of stress eating and boredom snacking hand in hand with the enforced inactivity due to lockdown regulations. A survey of more than eight hundred UK adults concluded that respondents had found it 'very' difficult to manage their weight during the pandemic with subjects recording anywhere between 3 and 15 pounds' weight gain in the six months following national restrictions.[6]

A glance back at the top Google search trends for 2020 confirms further still a shift in our priorities, with dieting, health, exercise and weight management searches near non-existent and replaced instead with 'How to cut men's hair at home?', 'Joe Biden', 'Covid testing near me' and 'protests near me'.

The world does not need another diet book ...

... A strange statement you might think, given the title of this book. The majority of modern diet books are filled with 'secrets', new discoveries and quick-fix guides to change your life and 'give you the body you've always dreamt of'. The reality however is that most consumers become the latest victim of a highly sophisticated marketing machine that feeds on our insecurities about our physical appearance. These marketing machines claim that *only* this book, these vitamins, those fat burners or that Ab Rocket 5000 can free your untapped self-obsessed potential and achieve what you really desire: the adoration and validation of others. It should be made clear that aiming for and Achieving goals of any kind is commendable. Tales of successful (and often extreme) weight loss are somewhat of an anomaly online in that they don't attract the kind of trolling that other content does, and that broadly, the fact someone has taken it upon themselves to change their life for the better and succeeded sets an un-questionably positive and important example. And yet, when compared to the sheer number of overweight people, especially in the western world, hometown stories of dramatic weight loss transformations are at best outliers, and in no way evidence of a communal acceptance that weight gain is dangerous in and of itself.

The diet book and fitness industry narratives are polarising. You would be forgiven for thinking that the world is split 50–50 into two key categories of people. The first 50 per cent are armed at all times with a protein shake and in between discussions about macros and training splits, pose for revealing selfies, which often leave little to the imagination. The second 50 per cent are gigantic sedentary land whales who spend their time either eating pizza or ordering it. Again, whilst these categories do exist, they are reflective of a tiny percentage of the population and the reality is that most people are smack bang in between these two vanishing points. For the centre majority, most of us carry more weight than we would like, and as lifestyle habits – such as long working hours, alcohol consumption and processed (often fast) food staples – catch up with us, our waistlines will continue to expand, adding on average 0.68kg (1.5lbs) of body fat per year. So, between the ages of 25 and 60 we can expect to gain 22kg (48.5lbs) of fat as a bare minimum!

It is this 'inevitable' adulthood weight gain that is the target of this book. This is not about looking good in your swimming trunks (as exciting as this may sound). This is why we say again that the world does not need another diet book. But what we do think it needs is an account of *why* adult weight gain is so pervasive and *how* far-reaching its effects are into every part of our lives. The world is in the throes of an obesity epidemic but the carrying of excess weight is not just weighing you down. It's killing you. Being overweight is either directly or a proxy of almost all preventable illness, nearly all cancers, chronic diseases and premature deaths.

The art of achieving and maintaining a stable healthy weight therefore, is not only desirable, but essential for living a healthful life, unhindered by costly prescriptions, medications and hospital visits for completely avoidable conditions.

This book is about the critical reasons why you must get your weight under control and not about the vanity metrics or the pursuit of getting washboard abs. In the chapters that follow, and in the classic style of the STOP series, we will first outline in Part One a simple guide to the science behind why we gain weight which will help you understand the risk factors that apply to you and get to grips with the cause-and-effect mechanisms at play. We will then share with you in Part Two simple-to-follow daily steps that will help you stabilise your weight, safe in the knowledge of why it is so critical that you do.

PART ONE

The Foundations

1

What is Energy Balance?

To understand how we gain weight we must first understand a critical mechanism of how the body works. In other words, how it is able to store heat to maintain basic bodily functions (a beating heart, inhaling and exhaling lungs, and eyesight, for example). The heat we need to sustain human life comes from the energy contained in food. This energy is known as ... you've guessed it ... calories. A calorie in its simplest form is a unit of measurement that describes the amount of heat needed to raise the temperature of one gram of water by 1 degree Celsius. Confused? We don't blame you. It never ceases to amaze us that a word so common is so rarely understood.

It's helpful to think instead of your body as having a pay-as-you-go electricity meter attached to it. The meter needs to be topped up each day with a bare minimum of say fifty English pence (50p) otherwise the body will switch off. You must maintain a daily feed of 50p pieces to sustain an optimal state where your brain, muscles, indeed every cell in your body is energised. Replace the coins with foodstuffs and you will now grasp the basic mechanism at play for why food is so important – it provides calories to sustain life. This is a process called 'energy homeostasis'.[7]

It logically follows from this that the body operates on a simple process of energy expenditure. The body needs a certain amount of energy to function, we consume calories, and then the energy is spent throughout the day by activity. This is more colloquially known as 'calories in – calories out' but, if we are going to be exact, it should really be 'energy in – energy out'. The body will either oxidise (use) what you eat or store the fuel you feed it. The point we should all be aiming for is when we oxidise the optimum amount of energy we need while avoiding any excess storage. This is the point of true energy balance, and you will be able to achieve energy balance yourself with the very straightforward routines in Part 2 of this book.

Metabolism

One's metabolism, simply put, is the processes of converting (metabolising) calories into energy. So if a calorie is a store of energy (the 50p), the metabolism acts as a refinery to process the components of the calorie and make available new energy for the body to use (the electricity meter).

It has long been agreed that men and women need a certain number of calories or amount of energy to operate a healthy body. This base level expectation is known as the Basal Metabolic Rate or BMR. Consuming significantly fewer calories than one needs is, therefore, the same as having *less* energy than your BMR requires for healthy bodily function. This results in an inability to perform basic human tasks, effectively resulting in significant fatigue, nutrient deficiency, a weakening of the bones, often irreversible impact to the immune system[8] and ultimately death.

Consuming far more calories than the body needs then is the same as having *more* stored energy than your BMR requires. A similar scenario happens across the fish industry all the time, with fishermen dumping tons of fish overboard because they have exceeded their quota. Or similarly, the 'flaring' protocol of the oil and gas industry, where surplus product is set on fire to maintain an exact amount of storage. Unfortunately, the body does not naturally opt to shed excess energy in such ways and instead stores any surplus as fat.

Fat has not always been the pantomime villain it is today. A study of human evolution shows that the consuming of excess calories for fat storage was not just tactical, but critical to the survival of early man. Periods of famine or harsh winters and other moments of predictable hunger meant that man could go for extended periods without eating and instead use these fat reserves for energy. This meant that even a lean adult male who weighs approximately 75kg (165lbs) could expect to store 100,000 kilocalories (kcal) of energy in reserve,[9] a process which has allowed man to survive for millions of years. Fat storage then is actually a pretty wonderful thing.

Primary energy groups

Conventional wisdom tells us that adult males need 2500 calories of energy per day while women require 2000 calories a day. The differential is due to the fact that adult males will typically weigh more and carry more muscle and therefore need slightly more energy invested to maintain proper bodily function. As we will discuss in Chapter 2, generalisations about the number of calories people need can be helpful when aiming to balance energy and maintain healthy weight. They are however often too vague, and don't clearly enough take into account age and activity ranges for people to action the insights and be consistent.

Staying with convention for now though, in order to maintain a healthy energy balance (energy in – energy out), mapping out how much you need to consume is, on the face of things, very straightforward. There are three primary food groups that we are sure you are very familiar with, each playing a critical role in maximising energy stores in the most optimum way, and a mix of these three components – carbohydrates, fats and proteins – is what is often described as a 'balanced diet'.

Carbohydrates

The first of these components is carbohydrates. The modern human has a brain far larger than other primates, and one which is very thirsty when it comes to the share of dietary energy it requires.[10] A carb is defined as containing carbon, hydrogen and oxygen in a ratio of 1:2:1.[11] Food that contains these compounds are digested far quicker than either fats or protein once they hit the engine room of the metabolism. For this reason, carbs are considered the primary source of energy for the body.

When people eat foods containing carbohydrates, the digestive system breaks them down into sugar.[12] This sugar enters the blood stream, providing a constant flow of energy through the body. Foods high in carbohydrates include pasta, beans, potatoes, rice and cereals.

In theory a 'carb is a carb' and for the purpose of understanding the mechanisms involved at this stage we will follow convention in describing them as such. However, in Chapter 8 we will discuss how not all carbohydrates are created equal, and the pursuit of true energy balance involves considering simple versus complex carbohydrates.

Fats

Dietary fat has become a very dirty word, in large part thanks to the fitness industry concluding that eating fat makes you fat. Without sufficient understanding of the roles of dietary fats it's fair to see why. Fats however play a critical role in energy balance and returning to and maintaining a healthy weight. The diet industry backdrop is incredibly unhelpful, and actually highly unhealthy, as it can make the scientific facts seem counter-intuitive. It is marketing folklore and now it seems common knowledge that fat will 'clog the arteries', which affects most notably the heart and the brain. The truth is however that just like carbohydrates and protein your body *needs* fats to absorb energy, but moreover it is needed to *protect* the heart and ensure optimum brain health. A 2018 study found that a diet too low in metabolised fats severely affected cognitive processing speed, emotions and the behaviour of the test subjects and concluded that dietary fats play a crucial role in optimum brain function.[13]

The anomaly here is that not all fats, just like carbs, are created equal. In Chapter 8 we therefore discuss exactly which fats should be part of your daily energy balance routine and which should not (including those which should perhaps be completely avoided).

Proteins

Protein is perhaps the most understood primary energy group and, on the whole, is accurately represented in both fitness and diet industry publications and content houses. Adequate consumption of dietary protein is critical for maintenance of optimum health and energy balance during normal human growth and ageing.[14] Protein contributes mainly to distributing energy for the purposes of maintaining lean body mass or of course building lean muscle through a process of enhanced remodelling and repair of the existing muscle.[15] In short, protein intake allows the micro tears within a person's muscles to regrow larger and stronger each time. Again, it is unsurprising that protein controls the conversation around body sculpting and body building, although these are not exactly prime examples of optimum energy balance at all.

Unlike carbohydrates and fats, protein sources are less complicated and as we will see in Chapter 8 there are numerous and plentiful sources to get your muscle energy fix.

2

The Basics of Energy Balance

Now that we've got an understanding of what energy balance is, we can look at how we can achieve energy balance in our diet. Helpfully, carbs, fats and proteins provide a fixed amount of energy (kcal) per gram of weight, which makes balancing your energy intake very straightforward.

Group	Energy (per gram)
Carbohydrates	4
Fats	9
Proteins	4

As we have shown, the primary energy groups each play an important role in maintaining energy balance so, in theory, the most effective method would be to follow a formula to achieve energy balance which takes the adult energy need and then divides it by 3.

2500kcal ÷ 3 = 833kcal per energy group
2000kcal ÷ 3 = 666kcal per energy group

Therefore, you would need to consume:

Men (2500kcal)	
Carbs	208g
Fat	92.5g
Protein	208g

Women (2000 kcal)	
Carbs	166g
Fat	74g
Protein	166g

When we eat above these amounts, we store that energy in reserve and begin to haul around extra weight, as the body goes into survival mode assuming that at some point in the near future these reserves will become depleted. But if the behaviours of the last century are anything to go by, for the majority (at least in the West) the hunger never comes and we enter prolonged energy storage, and that is being overweight defined.

So if it is seemingly so easy to reach energy balance, why do two thirds of us fail to do so? Chapters 4 and 5 will explore some of these stumbling blocks in detail, but by far the most basic reason we struggle is the assumed energy-need figures themselves (2500 and 2000 for men and women, respectively). It might seem counter-intuitive that there would be a blanket universal requirement for every adult man or woman, and that's because there isn't. The science of total energy needed is as diverse as the people and communities that need it. We know for certain that athletes, weightlifters, marathon runners and sportspeople eat higher volumes of food because they need more energy to fuel their higher rate of activity, and to heal, repair and build future muscle to increase their performance. Yet all too often we fail to consider that the same thing is true of the bus driver, the stay-at-home parent or the office worker – and of course the plethora of further deviations within the members of these defined groups. One bus driver might be largely sedentary while another climbs mountains in their spare time, for example.   The 2500/2000 energy split therefore, while well intentioned and generally well below the average energy consumed, is an unhelpful and confusing guide.

Finding YOUR Basal Metabolic Rate (BMR)

You will, we are afraid, have to come to terms with the fact that the success of this book comes from *you*, the reader's input, and not magically from this book's pages if left unapplied. You will be asked for effort and proactivity, but you will be amazed at the expediency of the rewards. We don't mean to put you off, but it does surprise us how severely intention outweighs results. The truth is, if you want to look like an athlete you must train and eat like an athlete. Equally, if you want to achieve energy balance to reverse the damage of weight gain and live an active, full, healthy and unabridged life you must calculate the BMR that relates specifically to you.

So, the task we are going to ask you to do is to calculate your own BMR right now. This is very straightforward, so please take a moment to work through the instructions below to work out your exact energy requirement. Once you have done so, please add it to the '6-Week Energy Balance Log' on pages 77–78 and continue reading.

The BMR Equation

On the following pages we are going to walk you through each equation for calculating your own BMR. This gives you an accurate guide to the amount of daily energy you need to be eating in order to achieve balance and prevent weight gain. The calculation is very easy and needs some basic apparatus which, if you don't have at home, we are sure you will be able to source directly, either from friends or by visiting your high street's pharmacy, which will have digital measuring tools free to use. You will need:

- Body weight scales (analogue or digital)
- Measuring tape
- Calculator
- Pen/pencil
- 6-Week Energy Balance Log (see page 77)

Using the equipment above, calculate the data points below:

A) 10 × your body weight in kilograms
B) 6.25 × your height in centimetres
C) 5 × your age

Now, put the data points into the following equation to get your specific BMR and note that there is a slight difference in equation for men and women.

$$\text{Men: } A + B - C + 51 = BMR$$
$$\text{Women: } A + B - C - 161 = BMR$$

Example:
A 45-year-old woman is 168cm (5'6") tall and weighs 75kg (165lbs) and the following data points are calculated as shown below.

A) 10 × 75 = 750
B) 6.25 × 168 = 1050
C) 5 × 45 = 225

$$750 + 1050 - 225 - 161 = 1414$$

We quickly see the exact amount of energy this woman needs every day is 1414 calories. As you may have already realised, if the woman in question was following the universal guidance of 2000 calories a day, she would be storing surplus energy and be out of balance to the tune of 586 kcals a day. In this example the woman is perhaps completely unaware that she is gaining significant weight by following seemingly clear health guidelines. Just shy of half a kg in body weight is equal to 3500 calories, so by adding almost 2kg a month in stored energy to her reserves, which will be converted into fat, could mean as much as 24kgs (over 50lbs) average weight gain per year! This is the equivalent of adding a small bale of hay, an average male bulldog or 27 litres (6 gallons) of water to the waistline every 12 months.

Fortunately, the reality is (slightly) less extreme, as BMR in its truest sense is the amount of energy your body needs for proper bodily function at rest and does not consider one's daily activity such as walking, talking and exercise. The National Academy of Sports Medicine tells us that true BMR measures energy expenditure in subjects reclining in a darkened room after 8 hours of sleep and following a 12-hour fast.[16] As much as the popular show *My 600-lb Life* would have you believe that this level of activity is not too far from the truth, we are certain that 99 per cent of people, including the woman in the example, are doing at least some daily activity by walking, driving, shopping or even washing. Therefore, in Chapter 6 we go into the next level of detail and calculate your True Basal Metabolic Rate (TBMR) so that you know exactly how much energy you need when considering the advised levels of activity and quickly achieve energy balance.

Before we get into these specifics we hope that the point here is clear. That even when studiously following the general health advice around daily recommended calories needed, the majority of people are over-consuming and slowly (and often not so slowly) gaining weight. But why is this such a problem? Why should you care if you carry extra weight? People of all sizes live long lives, so if I'm not body conscious can't I just continue to store energy I never use and not change my deeply held habits? These are all good questions, so in the next chapter we are going to discuss the harsh reality of why you must stop gaining weight today.

3

Why is Being Big a Big Deal?

It is interesting that when you are searching for information around maintaining healthy weight online there is a clear trend in advice around the benefit of reducing risk. Risk of heart attack, strokes and diabetes to name a few, so the research focuses on a reduction of risk, because it assumes, quite rightly, that a majority of people are at risk. A common behaviour is for people to search and research for advice reactively, so the lion's share of searches relating to health and fitness yield results such as 'quick transformations', 'lose fat fast' or 'regaining your youth'.

We want to turn this on its head and instead of looking at what makes you unhealthy, outline exactly what it means to be in optimum, balanced health.

What does healthy look like?

The World Health Organization (WHO) tells us that optimum health is a state of complete physical, mental and social wellbeing and not just the absence of disease or infirmity.[17] If you think this is vague, so do we. When we think about optimum health we generally conjure up images of lean individuals in activewear following energetic pursuits, or sportsmen and women competing in their craft. These are without doubt examples of healthy lifestyles, but they are more accurately a by-product of optimum health. Beauty, they say, is skin deep, but balanced health is far deeper still and while there are many leading indicators of good health, they all stem from proper energy balance with three fundamental mechanisms:

1 The Brain
2 The Cardiovascular System
3 The Lungs

Yes, rippling muscles and low body fat percentages are evidence of someone that has reached energy balance, but under the surface all roads lead back to the three fundamental mechanisms, as we shall show now.

The Brain

The adult brain is comprised principally of water, accounting for 75 per cent of its average 1.3-kilogram weight. It is home to approximately 100 billion neurons that process and transmit information of all kinds using electrical signalling.[18] This means that brain health is an energy-intensive exercise, controlling everything from our thoughts, memory and speech to movement of our arms and legs and the hard drive for the function of our organs and nervous system.[19] Normal brain function is highly dependent on an adequate supply of energy to perform these tasks. Again, energy is delivered in the form of consumed calories which are turned into sugars by the metabolism and delivered to the brain via the bloodstream. The brain is the body's command centre and it is in a constant process of resource allocation, so in addition to sufficient energy, the brain relies on one further element to function: oxygen, and plenty of it. Without it, the command centre cannot signal efficiently where to allocate blood around the body. It is therefore essential that a cerebral energy and oxygen supply chain exists to support the brain and body functions and this process is outsourced to the cardiovascular system.

The Cardiovascular System

It is a common misunderstanding that cardiovascular exercise relates to the lungs, when in fact it is derived from the words 'cardio' meaning 'heart' and 'vasco' meaning 'veins'. We suspect that the source of confusion is the heavy breathing associated with running or intensive exercise. The critical role of ferrying energy and oxygen to the brain is fulfilled by a massive network of blood vessels, the blood itself and the heart.

Blood vessels run through the entire body and form a natural highway for blood to carry nutrients, gases and hormones to and from cells. This highway is so extensive that if you were to lay it out end to end it would stretch 60,000 miles.[20] Yes, you read that correctly. There are enough arteries, capillaries and veins in your body right now to stretch 2.4 times around the Earth.

If the vessels are the road, then the blood is the workhorse, a living fluid which, because of its 55 per cent plasma (a light yellow liquid which helps to remove waste from cells) and 45 per cent formed elements (red and white blood cells and platelets), is more accurately described as fluid connective tissue[21] and not a simple fluid in and of itself. As its function is so critical, blood is abundant through the body and weighs in at 5 litres (1.2 to 1.5 gallons), around 10 per cent of an adult's body weight. Without sufficient pressure, however, and a mechanism to keep the blood flowing, gravity would pull all the blood down, pooling at the lowest point in the body.[22] This is a process known as 'lividity' and something that happens in the hours after we die. A macabre thought indeed, but luckily the vast network of the veins is a closed tube system in which the blood is propelled around these many miles by a muscular heart.[23]

If popular culture is to be believed, the heart is a somewhat flimsy organ worn carelessly on the sleeves of adolescents and when not being the target of winged naked babies armed to the teeth with a bow and arrows, is resigned to the categories of either 'achy' or 'breaky'. The reality is far from these *types of* anecdotes. If the brain is the command centre, the heart is without doubt the engine room, continuously pumping the equivalent of 9000 litres (2000 gallons) of nutrient-dense blood a day, or 5.6 litres per minute, to sustain life.[24]

In his 2000 article for the Wellness Institute and Research Center at Old Dominion University, David P. Swain likens the heart to the operation of a city water pump, which is used to pump fresh water up into a water tower from a river and into a network of pipes that lead to the surrounding township.[25] This is a simple analogy that clearly outlines the fact that without a pump (the heart), the remaining infrastructure is made redundant.

It is clear how gargantuan the task of the cardiovascular system is then, and also the multifaceted role it plays in energy and oxygen delivery. This brings us on to the final component of true optimum health, without which none of the pre-described processes and mechanisms would work.

The Lungs

The main function of the lungs is perhaps obvious in that it performs the essential role of respiration (or breathing). Respiration is the process of drawing in oxygen from the air into the blood, while at the same time expelling the harmful carbon dioxide and other waste gases. Total lung capacity in adults is about 6 litres[26] and each of us performs this gas exchange process through over 6 million[27] breaths a year. Much like the veins, the magnitude of the lungs' true size is not immediately obvious, and yet if you were to stretch all the complex components of the lungs out, they would cover around the size of a tennis court.

If the lungs were unable to work effectively or impaired, insufficient quantities of oxygenated blood would flow through the circulation to the brain and to all the other areas which rely on an adequate flow to thrive, such as the liver, the heart itself and the muscles.

When we put together all three components, we find an infinite chicken and egg loop – a harmonic relationship which is the bedrock of true balanced health, where each organ operates in perfect unison with the other. But isn't there a litany of other organs that contribute to optimum bodily function? In a single word, yes, however, without proper energy to fuel these critical areas the remaining beneficiaries can never reach true balance.

Losing your balance

It is vital that the narrative around optimum health is driven by this new context, where we think of good habits and health and their impact on the internal mechanisms and not just on the external indicators of health, which are all too often the focus. It cannot be underestimated that seeing health as only six-pack abs and low body fat is not just misguided, but lethal. The fitness industry will go to any lengths to portray debatably achievable yet desirable aesthetic results. The tactics behind the scenes such as steroids, fat burners, pills, powders and restrictive or force-feeding that the consumer does not see are the exact opposite of what is promised.

So, if we continue to overeat, over-store energy and gain weight, how does the process impact the three essential components of good health, what further consequences start to emerge and what are the invisible side effects of our habits which we only find out about when it's too late?

The Unbalanced Brain

The effects of weight gain on a balanced brain start to occur rapidly, principally in that all regions of the brain slow down essential activity and blood flow.[28] Reduced brain activity can result initially in low-level losses in concentration and knowledge (or memory) retention, but can extend to far-reaching effects in areas such as the prefrontal cortex – the area of the brain responsible for complex thinking, problem-solving, and self-control.

This cognitive effect can be gradual and is often dismissed as part of the ageing process, when in fact a secondary process is also at play, because being overweight affects the physical size of the brain too. Several studies have concluded that those with high levels of energy storage (excess body weight) show signs of cerebral atrophy[29] – the reduction in the size of brain cells, organ or tissue after attaining its mature growth. This makes key regions of the brain, such as the frontal lobes (responsible for language, emotion and sexual behaviour), temporal lobes (which preserve consciousness and long-term memory) and the hippocampus (which regulates motivation and learning) downgrade significantly.

You may be pre-empting the conclusion here that, along with the significant reduction in one's quality of life for a number of years, the final destination of an unbalanced brain is irreversible memory loss, dementia and potentially Alzheimer's disease. We often think of cognitive diseases as a natural part of ageing, but this is nonsense, and have now concluded that dementia and Alzheimer's are primarily 'lifestyle diseases' and that except for those with certain genetic predispositions are completely preventable. The staggering result of a poll conducted by Saga of 9000 over-50-year-olds, found that dementia was by far the most feared condition, outweighing the worry of cancer, stroke and heart conditions.[30] The fear of being unable to remember our family members, losing our home and independence and the isolation this would result in, outweigh fears of open-heart surgery and chemotherapy by 2:1. And yet the research tells us that adults who are overweight are at the most risk of dementia[31] but two out of three adults are still obese.[32] *

Finally, don't be fooled into thinking that cognitive decline from being overweight is the vanguard of the elderly. Dementia UK defines early onset dementia as diagnosed in those under the age of 65 and there are 42,000 people in this category today in the UK alone, with numerous cases of patients in their 30s and even early 20s.

Optimum brain health declines as it is unable to get an adequate flow of resources in the form of oxygen and energy through the blood. So, what is happening further down the supply chain to prevent the command centre from getting what it needs?

* You might be asking yourself 'But what about people who have genetic reasons for gaining weight?' The aim of the STOP series is to deal with the science as it applies to the majority of cases, and not to consider at length rare edge cases that, whilst important, might deter members of the general population who would benefit from the simple strategies presented.

The Unbalanced Cardiovascular System

To understand how being overweight effects the cardiovascular system is to understand the nuances of fat storage and the types of fat that the body metabolises excess energy into. As we know, excess energy is not expelled without intervention such as balanced energy intake based on your TBMR and is instead stored as fat in two key ways.

Subcutaneous fat, as the etymology suggests, sits 'sub' (under) 'cutaneous' (relating to the skin) and is the layer we pull and prod in front of the mirror. There should always be at least a prime layer of subcutaneous fat as it serves an important role to cushion deep tissue from external impact and blunt trauma.[33]

Figure I shows the typical locations of subcutaneous fat for both men and women, commonly referred to as the 'problem areas'. Both men and women store subcutaneous fat on their thighs, but it is more prevalent in the belly and 'love handles' for men, and the neck, breasts, arms and hips for women. Fat of this kind is a useful leading indicator as to the overall health of your body and whether or not you are achieving true energy balance. These are also the areas which will signal successful weight loss, and regular measurements of the waist, for example, is a good guide for progress.

While subcutaneous fat is necessary, carrying too much of it is problematic for several reasons. Firstly, subcutaneous fat is closely associated with insulin resistance, the name given when body cells don't respond properly to insulin.[34] This means that the sugars (glucose) that are processed by the metabolism cannot be distributed effectively, resulting in glucose build-up in the blood which is what we call high blood sugar levels. This can lead to a number of metabolic syndromes that leave the metabolism unable

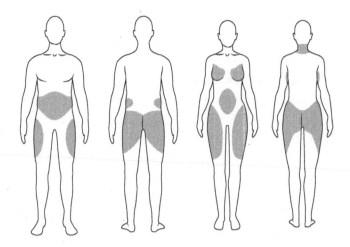

Figure 1: Distribution of subcutaneous fat in males and females

to conduct its essential duty, resulting in the body staying in a highly inflammatory state. Inflammation in the body can play an essential role in fighting off foreign invaders, such as parasites and bacteria that would otherwise make us sick, but being overweight causes the body to be in a *constant* state of inflammation. Cells become stressed as they respond to attacks that don't actually exist and then they start to become damaged, meaning healthy cells, organs and tissue can begin to scar and break down leading to severe conditions such as blindness, cancer and mental illness.[35]

Given that general health and fitness is almost exclusively focused on and interested in 'losing' subcutaneous fat, it is unsurprising that these problem areas are at the front of the mind for most people looking to lose weight and the reason for the majority of body-conscious insecurities. It follows that excess subcutaneous energy storage is closely associated with depressive illness, with a study from 2017 showing that 71 per cent of women experience generalised anxiety disorder as a direct result of their weight[36] which they feel, quite understandably, is at odds with society's projections of beauty. A further sting in the tail is that depressive disorders themselves are a key factor in comfort eating and gaining weight, which can all too often become a deadly catch-22 situation.

But what has all of this got to do with the cardiovascular system? we hear you ask. Subcutaneous fat can clearly be very concerning in and of itself, and you must follow the guide in Part 2 to map out your TBMR and achieve energy balance to prevent it. However, the actual concern around subcutaneous fat is that it is a leading indicator of the existence of a far more dangerous fat that lurks deeper. High levels of stored subcutaneous fat always points to the existence of visceral fat.

Visceral, or abdominal fat, is of particular concern as it sits around the organs themselves so, unlike subcutaneous fat that you can (and probably often do) grab with your hands, visceral fat lies out of reach deep in the abdominal cavity.[37] Fat that

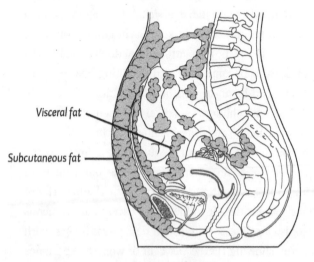

Figure 2

collects around the organs causes the arteries – part of the blood vessel network supply of energy and oxygen around the body – to stiffen and become harder. As the arteries lose their natural flex it becomes harder for the heart to pump blood through the supply chain, which raises the pressure of the blood, resulting in high blood pressure or hypertension. Think about how one might raise the pressure of a slow-flowing garden hose. When you obstruct the natural flow with your thumb, the pressure of the water instantly rises and what was moments ago a pathetic trickle can become a powerful jet. The problem is your arteries are not a garden hose and the consequences here are the building blocks for numerous serious and life-threatening health conditions.

This loss in blood vessel elasticity means that the heart must work much harder to pump blood around the body. Now that the blood flows far less freely a person may well start to experience chest pains which we call angina as well as noticing an irregular beat as the heart struggles to maintain enough per minute pumps for regular and healthy flow. Much like lifting weights forces your muscles to tear, repair and grow larger, this extra stress on the heart causes the organ itself to thicken and become far less efficient which marks the onset of heart disease and is a primary cause of heart attacks. In the UK alone, 4 million men and 3.6 million women currently live in this state.[38]

This story does not end well, as with continued pressure on the heart, and after what can be multiple heart attacks across a person's life time, we all too often find ourselves at the point of total heart failure with 450 people in UK per day succumbing to the disease.[39]

We have now come full circle, and while not one of the three critical organs affected by weight gain supersedes another, it could be argued that without the next organ the rest of the journey would not be possible, as sufficient energy flow is one thing, but the body can last only a matter of minutes without oxygen.

The Unbalanced Lungs

As we have discussed, without the lungs oxygenating the blood to give life to the organs, life does not last very long at all. We attack our respiratory system with many lifestyle habits and extracurricular activities, most notably smoking, but we don't often understand how being overweight alone has equally concerning effects. In fact, as the rates of weight gain increase worldwide so too do clinical presentations of many respiratory diseases.[40] And aside from serious cases resulting in death, there are numerous related diseases that millions of people endure for life completely unaware that their over-stored energy is a primary cause of, most notably, asthma.*

The mechanisms at play here are very straightforward. As you increase your weight, you increase the amount of stored energy around the chest, which compresses the diaphragm (the muscle that contracts when we breathe), the lungs and the chest cavity itself. An accumulation of visceral fat around the abdomen affects the downward movement of the diaphragm and chest. Added together, these processes result in significantly lowered functional lung volume,[41] or the minimum amount of air the lungs should be able to draw into the body to meet the minimum expectation of oxygenated blood needed for balanced health.

Lung function will of course decline over time and is an unfortunate by-product of ageing, as cells lose their ability to

---

* We refer here to chronic or onset asthma, which can develop at any time in one's life well up to and beyond the age of 50, rather than any genetic pre-disposition.

respawn as efficiently and as vigorously as they once did. However, a 2020 study conducted over a 25-year period concluded that 100 per cent of the participants that were unable to maintain an energy balance accelerated the rate their lungs declined at and that weight-related lung disease itself should be considered an epidemic and a powerful predictor of morbidity in the general public.[42] Interestingly, lung decline was also shown in participants with only moderate weight gain, not just in the more extreme cases as we often like to assume. A second study found that it was also not just adults who were at risk, and that early signs that your lungs are beginning to decline, shortness of breath and wheezing, were as common in young adults and children. Rapid early weight gain has become far too common and is characterised by wheezing illnesses in early life leading to lower function and quality of life in childhood.[43]

In summary, it is easy to see how increased weight affects the three core building blocks of balanced health. You will note there has been no mention of aesthetic implication or athletic performance, as the true consequences of gaining weight are far more fundamental, but criminally under-discussed in the popular narrative around why one should balance one's energy. This has nothing to do with looking good for summer and everything to do with living actively for as many summers as possible.

As alarming as we hope this chapter has been, there is some good news to end on. Reversing the effect of weight-gain-related issues in the three core regions is, if not easy, very straightforward. The body is a highly responsive machine and it is itching to regain its optimum balance and health as long as you are willing to follow the steps in the second part of this book. Please do not take stories of rapid reversal lightly though, and conclude that action can wait for another day, week or month. You simply cannot afford to continue putting strain on your essential mechanisms, and yes, complete return to health is possible with proactivity, but it can equally become irreversible if left to a rainy day.

4

Pervasive Myths

Stigma around weight is a cause of great distress for millions of people and cyberbullying has become commonplace. Pop star Jessie Nelson, a 28-year old, describes how she 'starved herself for weeks' and attempted suicide following remarks made about her weight by a number of tabloid news pundits.[44] With the backdrop of 46 per cent of Britons feeling 'unhappy or very unhappy about their weight',[45] it would seem that this issue will get worse before it improves, especially as obesity worldwide triples every 25–30 years. The root cause here is that people generally worry, or are unhappy about their aesthetic appearance and the effect that weight gain has from the outside looking in. And perhaps not without good reason. A study showed that first impressions count for a lot, as after a workplace survey half of employers were reported to be less inclined to recruit obese candidates, citing the assumptions that with visibly excess weight comes less motivation, less self-discipline and less competence.[46] Snap judgements are unhelpful and undoubtedly lead to many employers losing out on great and diverse talent flowing into their companies.

It is essential that this does not become a stigma however. As we have discussed, the facts are that people who store excess energy will, by definition, have reduced working lives. Why? Because the mechanisms at play guarantee they will have shorter lifespans. Period. And their quality of life beyond middle age will start to become a barrier to the working hours most cities now expect.

Once people understand that weight gain is not about aesthetic perfection (and we now know it couldn't be less about this) and is about true energy balance for optimum health and lifespan, we believe the conversation will change to one of support rather than stigma. Energy balance is really quite easy and achievable and it is within the remit of 99 per cent of people who are overweight or obese. But they must have the support to apply it and change their thinking around it.

Healthy at any size?

It is within this context that we discuss a concurrent narrative that is of equal concern to that of 'fat shaming' and weight stigma. The 'healthy at any size' movement. Body positivity has taken great strides in recent years and has spurred an industry that embraces all shapes and sizes and even the advent of the plus size male and female model on the catwalk. This is without question a good, no, great, thing and is the reason we don't at any point cite aesthetic outcomes as a reason to buy and action the advice in this book. Beauty does not fall into a narrowly defined box and whatever size a person is has no bearing on the millions of people that find them utterly irresistible. Beautiful at any size is without question, but the mantra that one can be healthy at any size is inexcusable, dangerous and kills more people than it empowers.

The Association for Size Diversity and Health (ASDAH) quite rightly 'celebrates bodies of all shapes and sizes' (although the first image on their website at the time of writing is a group of slim individuals raising a toast). But it goes on to challenge the empirical evidence around the consequences of weight gain and maintaining excess energy, and that its 'oppressed' members would benefit more from dismantling weight-centred health policies and practices. Indeed, ASDAH member Mckenna Schueler writes that we should look to combat harmful cultural messaging that glorifies weight loss, and instead reframe gaining weight as an act of self-care and body kindness.[47]

We are convinced that Schueler's remarks, and those of the cohorts of other healthy-at-any-size advocates are well intentioned and come from a genuine place of concern for those who endure weight-related stigma. However, we hope it is now obvious how potentially dangerous and counter-intuitive this messaging really is. We must as a world population come to terms with the fact that being overweight is very much not an ideal state and does, in every possible case, reduce life quality and life expectancy, and cause the death of its disciples.

This may come across as harsh or insensitive, which is not our intention. Obesity will continue to kill 2.8 million people worldwide per year, long after vaccine rollouts have taken place and public interest in the subject wains. And yet we are not regularly confronted with news about the end of times in light of the weight crisis even though it threatens 67 per cent of adults at the time of writing. It is important now, more than ever, to ensure that the activism of the ASDAH and others like it does not overtake this stark reality in favour of a narrative that honourably seeks diversity and inclusion, but ignores potentially fatal risks.

The connection between energy balance and cancer

In the wake of Covid-19, news sources waxed lyrical about the incidences of wrongly concluding a death was 'Covid related'. A 2020 article by Thompson Reuters claimed to have evidence that 94 per cent of the 153,504 official Covid deaths were in fact associated with other causes and that the real figure was closer to 9000 where Covid was the sole cause of deaths in the US up to that point.[48] This gives some credence to the popular internet meme that was circulating at the time which suggested that if you were eaten by a shark, and the autopsy showed you were positive for coronavirus then this was clearly ... a Covid-related death. The facts in both cases, serious or not, have been heavily disputed and will no doubt be a source of contention for many years in the post-Covid world. However, it has raised an important understanding of 'comorbidity' or the existence of two or more conditions or illnesses in a patient at any one time.

This is the precise lens that should be used to understand the effects of weight gain, but it is rarely discussed or deemed significantly newsworthy. If we were to truly understand the impact here we suspect this might change, and quickly, given the consequences of inaction. Millions of deaths are categorised solely as caused by specific cancers or conditions when in fact they are actually weight gain related. A pooled study in 2005 found that 937 million adults in the world are overweight, and 396 million were obese. It also found that in the US, 85,300 new cancer cases occurred per year that were directly related to obesity.[49] A second study found that an increase in body weight accounted for a significant increase in overall cancer risk[50] and that there were at least 13 leading cancers for which being overweight is a significant contributing factor.

1. Oesophageal
2. Liver
3. Kidney
4. Stomach
5. Colorectal
6. Advanced prostate
7. Post-menopausal breast
8. Gallbladder
9. Pancreatic
10. Ovarian
11. Endometrial[51]
12. Myeloma
13. Meningeal

The statistics associated with these cancer types are alarming – a small snapshot of which is outlined below:[52]

- Women who are overweight are 40 per cent more likely to develop breast cancer
- Risk of gallbladder cancer increases by a factor of 60 per cent
- 1.5 times higher risk of pancreatic cancer
- Overweight people twice as likely to develop liver cancer
- 10 per cent increase in both ovarian and thyroid cancer
- Risk of slow-growing brain tumours (meningiomas) rises by 50 per cent
- Kidney cancer is doubled
- Colorectal cancer increases by 30 per cent
- Gastric cardia and oesophageal cancer are twice as common in overweight individuals
- Overweight women are 400 per cent more likely to develop endometrial cancer

Perhaps more tragic than these statistics is the fact that so many of these cancer cases are totally preventable and needless. A silver lining to this rather distressing story is that cancer risk can be reduced by as much 45 per cent in those who have reduced their stored fat back to balanced levels. If you are in a group that sits in a high cancer risk category because of your weight gain, you must without delay take the simple steps mapped out in Part Two and begin the process of reversing the mechanisms at play.

It goes without saying that even though an alarming number of conditions are associated with excess energy storage there are a host of others that are not directly linked but do form a more complete risk framework. With this in mind we will conclude Part One of this book with a discussion about compound habits.

5

Compound Habits

Compound habits refer to the habits and lifestyle choices that we all make which impact adversely on our health and wellbeing. A process that gains momentum significantly when we add them to the backdrop of consistent energy over-storage and weight gain. The primary habits we will discuss, that exacerbate energy imbalance, are:

- Sedentary lifestyle
- Smoking
- Drinking alcohol*
- Stress and long working hours

Sedentary lifestyle

Life in the modern era is defined by our ability to experience more than ever before without having to once leave the comfort of our living rooms. It is a strange paradox where we can travel without

---

* It is worth noting that soft drinks are also of equal concern, as they have a high number of calories which are useless for nutrition; but there is a link between their consumption and overeating.

the activity it would have once taken for us to get somewhere, and while an increase in knowledge is no bad thing, the risk-reward is starting to catch up with us.

Bingeing is a common pastime both in terms of the food we eat and now also in how we describe the amount of time we allocate to 'Netflix and chill', which is problematic for a number of reasons. Firstly, the unquestioned acceptance that most evenings will involve little to no exercise at all, replaced by 21 episodes of an infinite number of boxsets, TV series and films. The compound issue here is that all too often this entertainment is loaded with either paid promotion or regularly interrupted with advertising campaigns for soft sugary drinks, ice cream, potato chips and a swathe of fast, or now, restaurant-quality foods delivered to your door in 30 minutes. Any seasoned fan of *The Simpsons*, which has in the UK been broadcast daily between 6 and 7 p.m. for over a decade, will associate the Domino's pizza sponsorship adverts as a standard feature of the show.

Inactivity plus the temptation to consume high energy and nutritionally devoid foods is a disaster already well established. Harvard University found that alongside the promotion of unhealthy food and beverage choices, the associated weight gain was not only alarming but led to the exact opposite of the joy, happiness and contentment these products promise and instead was directly correlated to higher rates of depression and type-2 diabetes.[53]

A balanced life does not mean a life with no entertainment, downtime or even the occasional binge (in moderation). In Part 2 of this book we show you the simple daily steps you can take to ensure that you can kick back and watch the game or your favourite show guilt-free, but we also stress the importance of experiencing life beyond digital screens.

Smoking and vaping

We are sure you won't need reminding of the clear and present danger that smoking presents. The evidence is irrefutable and has probably impacted the lives of the majority of the readers of this book in some way already. Weight gain has overtaken smoking as the leading cause of preventable death in the UK, as successful campaigns and price hikes have led to fewer people taking up smoking as a habit. In the UK smoking still accounts for 19.4 per cent of overall deaths, which is a staggering figure for a habit that provides no benefits whatsoever. Interestingly, it has been found that being overweight is as hazardous to one's health as smoking 10 cigarettes a day, making a strong link between weight gain and premature death.[54]

As we discussed in Chapter 3, the pressure that visceral fat puts on the mechanics of the respiratory system, coupled with the serious effects that smoking has in exactly the same area can be seen without exaggeration as the perfect storm. Smoking damages the airways and leaves deposits in the arteries which clog and further aggravate veins that have already been stiffened by surrounding fat. This restricts steady and reliable blood flow to the heart and brain, hastening the decline into cardiovascular disease and ultimately heart attack and heart failure.

Luckily smoking is becoming less and less of an option for newcomers tempted to start, given the sky-high prices of buying a pack of cigarettes, but a burgeoning industry has grown exponentially over the last five years to take its place. Vaping promises the pleasure of smoking without the harmful chemicals associated with cigarettes and, on the face of things, this is true. Although the jury is still out on the harm that heating synthetic flavourings can have on the body, we can assume that the absence of toxins found in cigarettes such as arsenic, tar and formaldehyde is at least an improvement. Most vaping mixtures do still deliver a high dose of the additive nicotine however, and this highly addictive substance hooks the user into an unnecessary expense. The National Health Service in the UK does not recommend switching to vaping for this exact reason and promotes instead methods of complete cessation from nicotine.

It is important to note that Johns Hopkins Medicine references thousands of lung-related injuries and numerous deaths associated with vaping due to the impact that thickening agents in the e-liquids have on the respiratory system. As such, vaping, like smoking, is a concerning compound habit which people must avoid even if you are not overweight.

Drinking alcohol

We sense that we might lose a few hearts and minds with this section. Drinking alcohol has cultural significance around much of the Western, and large parts of the Eastern, world. It is the centrepiece of every celebration, condolence and any event in between ('event' is used loosely here, as 57 per cent of adults admit to drinking more than once a week).[55]

Many studies have argued that sensible alcohol consumption is safe and, in some cases, not healthy, but also not overly unhealthy. And while alcohol alone will on average kill 14.8 men and 6.9 women per 100,000 in the UK,[56] this is not the reason we have chosen to focus on booze as a compound habit. Put simply, if you're not eating excess calories, you're drinking them. Alcohol in its most popular forms (beer, wine, alcopops and mixed spirits) are high energy drinks packing masses of calories in relatively small portions. The average pint of lager weighs in at 227kcal with a large glass of white wine not far behind at 190kcal. In isolation these drinks can easily be factored into a healthy, energy-balanced lifestyle. However, on an average Friday and Saturday night most people can expect to drink a bare minimum of 3–4 drinks (with no real upper limit). Based on this unlikely minimum, the average beer drinker can expect to add at least 2000kcal in alcohol if they drink each weekend, which many do for much of the year. This unfortunately is not sustainable in an energy-balanced diet unless you are foregoing proper energy in food form to drink instead, which in Chapter 6 we will show is far from ideal.

The story does not end there either, as a standard habit of late-night food is still to come into play. Even modest portions of the nation's favourite post-pub snacks will add 1000–3000kcal in additional and unneeded energy which head straight for the stores in the form of subcutaneous and visceral fat. This is a compound habit defined, where massive amounts of excess calories are consumed on a regular basis under the banner of normal socialising.

We are not here to tell you to stop drinking – enjoying alcohol is not a bad habit in and of itself and can be a tool for positivity in helping people socialise or unwind. However, if you have really taken on board the message of this book so far (that excess energy is killing you) then we're afraid you cannot achieve energy balance and drink as described above. You simply can't have it both ways. We speak with patients all the time who can't bear even the thought of relinquishing what is a bone fide 'important part of their life', and we suspect that this is a view shared by many. Far from accepting this, we challenge you as we did them to think what a genuinely depressing statement this actually is, where your life is governed by a beverage, and which if left unchecked will take it all away.

Stress and long working hours

A 2018 study found that people who endure medium- to long-term elevated levels of stress had increased amounts of the hormone cortisol in their bloodstream.[57] Cortisol is known as the stress hormone and at adequate levels can play an important role in controlling blood sugar levels and regulating the metabolism. However, in higher quantities cortisol starts to raise the blood pressure, weakens the muscles and can cause rapid weight gain, especially around the abdomen. Elevated levels of cortisol are ironically linked closely with overeating, which has the obvious by-product of excess energy storage coupled with the fact that it also prevents the metabolism from operating properly and results in poorly distributed energy, and can store low calorie intake as belly fat.[58]

The advice is simple then. Stop being stressed? As you might guess it's not that easy, as according to the American Institute of Stress (AIS) 33 per cent of people report extreme stress and the remaining 77 per cent of people experience stress that affects their physical health.[59] It is now more important than ever to take steps to get your stress under control. We literally mean steps. In Part Two of this book we will discuss the many positive effects of base-level activity on your mental wellbeing and which will help to break your working day up and get you away from the desk (no phones allowed).

*

Gaining weight is no joke and is often the root cause of, or at least associated with, almost all preventable disease-related death. A deeper understanding of the mechanism of weight gain can help dispel the myths around dieting offered by the fitness and nutrition industry, and reconceptualising the problem as one not of fat, but of energy storage, and not of weight loss, but of energy balance can make the real path to success much more tangible.

We hope that Part 1 of this book has had a real impact and given you the understanding and drive to stop the damage of weight gain and achieve true energy balance. You're now ready for Part 2 where we will show you exactly how to achieve it.

PART TWO

What You Can Do

Notice:

If you have jumped straight to this section, then welcome! The mentality for a quick and easy fix is something we have anticipated, which is why the routines are not only short, but useable without reading any other element of this guide. However, achieving energy balance can only come from a sufficient awareness of the nuances of why we gain weight and the dangers of doing so. Please take a few moments to work through Part One before continuing to Part Two.

6

A Blueprint for True Energy Balance

Following the guidance from Chapter 3 you will have already calculated your Basal Metabolic Rate (BMR) and added it to the first page of the 6-Week Energy Balance Log on page 77. As we discussed in that chapter, the widely held and generic assertions about the amount of energy one needs are unhelpful and often work against energy balance, so the BMR calculation allows you to start the process of making this about you. Again, BMR only gives you the figure of your energy requirement when your body is at rest, so what we must now do is calculate what we call True Basal Metabolic Rate (TBMR). On a simple-to-follow sliding scale this will allow you to factor in the energy needed for basic activities, all the way up to, should you be so brave, heavy weekly exercise so that you are not over- or indeed under-fuelling your body.

As a recap, where A is 10 × your body weight in kg, B is 6.25 × your height in cm and C is 5 × your age, the BMR equation is as follows:

$$\text{Men: } A + B - C + 51 = \text{BMR}$$
$$\text{Women: } A + B - C - 161 = \text{BMR}$$

The TBMR equation asks you to take the BMR figure and multiply the total by the figure on the table below which best describes your current level of activity.

Activity Level	Description	TBMR
1 Little to non-existent	No exercise at all	TBMR = BMR × 1.2
2 Light (average)	Walking 1–3 times a week	TBMR = BMR × 1.375
3 Moderate	Sports or gym >3 a week	TBMR = BMR × 1.55
4 High	High intensity >5 a week	TBMR = BMR × 1.75
5 Extreme	Training twice a day	TBMR = BMR × 1.9

Without wanting to make snap judgements, the majority of people will likely find themselves in the top two levels of little to no exercise or light activity, apart from spontaneous yet short-lived periods of activity throughout the year, and particularly in January. Returning to the example in Chapter 3 of the 45-year-old woman who is 168cm (5'6") tall and weighs 75kg (165lbs), the BMR equation is:

$$750 + 1050 - 225 - 161 = 1414 \text{ kcal}$$

The woman is broadly inactive and has a 40-hour week desk job which resigns her to the little activity category. Her TBMR is therefore calculated as follows:

$$1414 \times 1.2 = 1697 \text{ kcal}$$

What's really interesting in this example is that only when she moves to the second category of light exercise, perhaps by walking to the shops rather than driving and doing errands on foot in local areas does she get close to the generic assumption of 2000kcal for women. In the absence of activity, she, as many others do, can follow the health guidance and steadily store energy day in day out.

This should also start to make you think back to the dangers of compound habits. It would not be unreasonable to assume that someone would have 2 glasses of wine every Friday and Saturday evening or at least 4.6 glasses spread across the week. At an average 190kcal per glass the 18.4 glasses drunk over the month would equate to an additional 3500kcal to the energy stores which, on top of the TBMR food intake requirement, would lead to an average weight gain of 0.5kg (1.1lbs) a month. It's pretty shocking to think that what would be considered perfectly sensible drinking habits will add 6kg (1 stone) to our waistlines every year.

Now it is time for you to calculate your own TBMR and please be honest with yourself. If you are not doing hill sprints twice a day, as much as you plan to, allocate your activity levels accurately. This is about what you do right *now* and as your energy and activity levels increase you can return to recalculate the TBMR and keep track on the TBMR log.

You will notice that the TBMR log asks you to enter a new TBMR every 6 weeks. Why? As you begin to balance your energy and start to redistribute and lose weight your TBMR will change and you must compensate. We did say that this process will take some commitment to follow correctly and it is essential that you do, as the TBMR you have today could mean you are over- or under-eating in a month's time. Staying with the example of the 45-year-old woman whose TBMR was 1697kcal of energy needed per day at a weight of 75kg. After 6 weeks she has shed a good amount of fat and is now 70kg and she has had a birthday in that time, but she is still doing little to no exercise. Her new TBMR will have changed as follows:

$$700 + 1050 - 230 = 1520 \times 1.2 = 1824 \text{ kcal}$$

TBMR can swing up and down person to person; in this case the loss of excess fat (and the potential increase in new lean muscle mass) has meant that the metabolism is working much more efficiently and is no longer slowing itself down, so it needs more calories to work optimally. This is good news for the lady as she can now add a further 127kcal per day to her diet and still maintain energy balance. A small glass of wine anyone?

The truth is that energy balance is something that we will have to monitor for the rest of our lives. There is no point pretending that this is a 90-day diet plan and then back to 15 pints on a Friday. It really is not much work, but has unrivalled benefits to your longevity and the amount of time your life is spent in good health and not hindered by preventable ailments. Having said this, there is no point doing this calculation daily, which you might well be tempted to do given the progress you will be making, but every 6 weeks is the advice. Firstly, you need the time to at least embed the habit of eating perhaps more tactically than you currently are, but more importantly we don't want you to become obsessed by the scales.

7

Raising the Activity Bar

If you are in Activity Levels 3–5 in the table, you will still find this chapter on activity a useful framework, but feel free to skip to Chapter 9 armed with your TBMR. For those residing in Activity Levels 1–2 however, it is important to put in place a system that allows you to easily raise your activity levels consistently to hasten energy balance and a whole host of additional benefits.

Step to victory

Walking is a staple of human activity and it is the bedrock of good health. And yet we have as a world population lost our way when it comes to moving around under our own steam. Whether it's the inclement weather in certain countries that means we opt for cabs over strolls in a cagoule, or the ease of home delivery, we are moving further and further away from the basic expected levels of activity for human beings. Gone are the days (for most) of walking miles to the next town for school or the nearest shop, and this is certainly progress, but getting a base minimum number of steps in a day has immediate benefits.

A Harvard Medical School study found that people in Activity

Level 1 – generally sedentary individuals confined to the home – would still do approximately 2500 steps a day, moving around the house. They concluded that increasing this to 4400 steps a day reduces mortality by 41 per cent[60] and this figure grows exponentially the more you are able to do it consistently every day. 10,000 steps a day has become somewhat of a gold standard in the health industry and equates to 7.6 kilometres (4.7 miles) a day or 53.2 (33 miles) a week, which is about the same as walking from Central London to Croydon and back again. While we would love readers to down tools and start walking 10,000 steps a day overnight, in reality the distance is not the blocker, as daunting as it might seem – it's actually the time. For a strong walker, 10,000 steps is over an hour a day commitment, but for the average person you are looking at closer to two hours. Whether or not you want to set 10,000 as a goal (and good on you if so) what we want to suggest instead is a gradual walking regime which you can easily implement and will help you rise through the activity levels and inform your TBMR.

Getting to Activity Level 1

For the first week we want to ease in gently those who are not used to walking so much. Keeping a record in your Walking Tracker beginning on page 80, the goal is to aim for a total of 77 minutes walking for the week. This equates to just 11 minutes per day. Please note that if you are not used to activity of this level you will experience some minor discomfort, particularly in your shins. This is totally normal and is just your body getting back into the swing of things.* You may also

---

* As this is very light exercise, you should not feel the need to consult a healthcare professional before adopting a walking regime. If at any time you start to experience severe pain, light-headedness or chest pains then please consult a doctor before

experience some mild soreness in the calves and thighs as the week passes; this is known as DOMS or delayed onset muscle soreness as your body is repairing itself and beginning to rebuild muscle in key areas to help you progress. Again, record your daily progress of Week 1 in the tracker, and if it helps, use the Notes section to reflect on how you felt, if something was easier or harder than you thought, or any random thoughts that popped into your mind as a result of time way from work and the screen. You are going to repeat this process for a second week.

By the beginning of Week 3, 11 minutes a day is going to seem like a doddle and you may have already started extending the walks out. This is great progress. Move your walking to 20 minutes a day for five days and if you can, challenge yourself to walk for 30 minutes on the sixth day (perhaps easiest on a weekend) followed by a day of rest. Follow this for a second week and you have advanced to Activity Level 2 and should now multiply your BMR by 1.375 to give you your new TBMR.

Getting to Activity Level 2

Activity Level 2 is defined by 35 minutes walking daily for five days. Remember, don't worry about the step count, this is about time spent on your feet, ideally outside, but a treadmill will have most of the benefits too.* This is followed by 60 minutes on the sixth day and a day of rest. At this level of activity, it is worth having a think about your walking technique and particularly your posture.

continuing.

* Treadmills do not require the same amount of energy as walking outside does, as the conveyer belt is doing some of the work for you in terms of leg propulsion. The variance in gradient and walking surfaces outside also improves coordination and provides a much more complete period of exercise in terms of targeted muscle groups and long-term injury prevention.

Being hunched over a desk, as many are these days will mean your natural resting position will have become more arched in the back. Counteract this by walking upright with your head above your shoulders. This is made easier by pushing your chest out like a robin. This will in turn cause some level of DOMs in the first week or so as your back muscles get reacquainted with the idea of supporting your weight. Log your activity in the Walking Tracker and again note down the nuances of the activity that apply to you and take a moment to reflect on the notes of the weeks prior and how far you have come in such a short amount of time.

This is the base level activity for Level 2. Increase the amount you walk or adopt supplementary activity such as cycling, swimming or stretching exercises to progress further to Level 3 if you are motivated to do so, and remember to factor this move into your TBMR calculation at the next 6-week interval.

Ditch the phone (or at least the work phone)

In Chapter 5 we spoke about the compound habit of stress and the debilitating effects it has on the mind and body. Elevated stress in most cases is work- or home-life related, with the former generally exacerbating the latter. With this in mind we would challenge you to do your daily walking without your phone. Leaving home without their lifeline might seem unfathomable for many people, but there is a wealth of evidence that shows how disconnecting for only a short time can reduce cortisol levels significantly. With the advent of smartphones, being out of the office or away from the desk does not necessarily mean being away from work, so at the very least ditch your work phone, and set work-associated apps to silent mode on your personal device while out walking.

We understand that many will use the time while out walking to reconnect with music, audio books, podcasts or mindful apps. This is of course fine, and in the weeks 1–4 especially, these can give you additional reason to get up and go. If you simply can't walk for 30 minutes without some kind of mind chewing gum helping you through it then don't worry, the walking should be your main priority. We would challenge you however to, at least twice a week, remove the headphones, put the phone on 'do not disturb' (or leave it at home) and walk with only your thoughts for company. This is the real process of detoxing your digitally controlled mind and will afford you a fixed amount of time a day to work through the factors in your life that cause you stress. A real, impactful moment of self-care which often allows you to resolve much of what is on your mind. Switch off, relax and repair.

8

Eating for Balance

It never ceases to amaze us that, through no fault of their own, one of the key reasons people gain weight is because they follow the advice and guidance from official associations. We have shown how problematic the advice from the General Medical Council is around general calorie intake, but the same is true for the types of food we are told support a balanced diet. As we shall discuss, there are simple tactics you can deploy to get back on track.

Turning the food pyramid on its head

The British Nutrition Council designed and implemented the UK government's 'Eat Well Guide', which is aimed at adults and for use in schools to make better sense of the conflicting information around health and nutrition.[61] The campaign centres on the primary energy groups and uses, as numerous other food- and health-governing bodies have done around the world; a summary of them in the form of a food pyramid looks something like the diagram overleaf.

This food pyramid shows food groups and the rough amounts that should be in one's diet, with grains and starchy carbohydrates

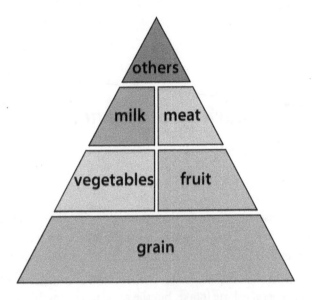

Figure 3: The food pyramid

accounting for most of the intake while proteins such as dairy and meat products, which they advise should factor less, just below junk food.

Now if the idea, as Figure 3 shows, that the basis of balanced nutrition is toast, muffins, waffles and cereal seems counter-intuitive, that's because it's wrong This diet structure may well have been ideal in the late 1800s to early 1900s when food supply and famine still ravaged much of Europe and so high calorie foods were a necessity, but in today's world, the food pyramid needs updating. Actually, it needs turning on its head.

As we outlined in Chapter 2 the principles of energy balance are very straightforward and holds that carbohydrates are needed in equal measure to protein. The pyramid as shown above is actually a pretty perfect blueprint to *gain* weight, not maintain it, with the lion's share of energy being provided by calorie-dense, nutritionally devoid foods, which are hard to not overeat.

Most modern cereals and grain-based foods are laden with all kinds of ingredients and often mark a perfect and deceitful balance between fat and sugar. Your brain is no fool and knows when it is eating too much of one kind of energy source and will take measures to make you put the fork down. Imagine trying to eat something very fat-dense like olive oil or butter. The amount of unaccompanied raw oil or butter you could eat would be very limited because your brain would quickly prevent you from overindulging. Ever heard someone say 'this brownie is too rich' or 'this sauce is too sweet'? This is that exact safety mechanism at work.

What the brain cannot do however is register when the combined energy profiles of fat and carbohydrates are put together in certain ways. Ever worked your way through an entire baguette smothered in French butter? Or eaten an entire cheese pizza? This is why you can. Your brain does not register the mountains of cheese, or masses of sugar in the dough as individual sources, which allows you to bypass the safety area and stuff your face. A study from Yale University found that the pairing of fat and carbs was also the primary trigger for food cravings and how in fact foods that are 'supra-addictive' elicit a sense of reward in your brain even if you don't like one of the components.

A proper food pyramid then should look more like an hour-glass where carbs and protein sit at opposite ends in equal measure with a layer in between that accounts for fats.

Good carbs, bad carbs, I know I've had my share

As mentioned earlier, there are two types of carbohydrates: complex and simple. In theory it does not matter which type of carb you consume to meet your energy-balance target; however, you should opt for complex carbohydrates and avoid most simple carbohydrates where possible. Simple carbs are categorised as those high in refined sugar or which act quickly and are metabolised almost instantly. A chocolate bar can give a temporary boost in energy but once the initial spike is gone the energy level drops back to where it was before, which now feels less than before you ate the bar. Whilst simple carbs occur naturally in fruits, vegetables and dairy products, those you should avoid are more commonly added to cakes, syrups, sweets, chocolate, soft drinks and alcohol, and do provide energy, but none of the fibre, vitamins or minerals you can expect from the whole food variants.

Bizarrely, simple carbs will take up more of your energy daily allowance more quickly, but with less volume, which has the run-off of leaving most people unsatisfied, or not satiated, and all the more likely to overeat or tempt you to indulge.

To bring to life what we mean, think of the energy available from sweets versus rice. A 55g bag of skittles has 222kcals of energy which is nearly all carbohydrate in the form of refined sugar. This could well be over 10 per cent of one's total energy need, and 50 per cent of the daily carb energy split. Skittles, and sweets like it, are not designed to relieve hunger, so the nutrition you gain is minimal, if not non-existent. Importantly, if you now compare this to an equivalent 222kcal of a complex carb like rice, you would be getting 200g of food, nearly four times the volume of the skittles, which are not metabolised instantly like a simple carb. Complex carbs instead release energy slowly over time, keeping you feeling satisfied, your energy levels steady and constant and all well within your daily allowance.

Staving off simple carbs and treats in the form of simple sugars completely is probably futile long-term and frankly unnecessary. The point here is you will struggle to maintain energy balance if you have simple carbs as a daily staple. Have them occasionally and always factor them into your TBMR total, and carbs, fats and protein split. Opt instead most of the time for complex carbs which are packed with essential nutrients, such as:

- Unrefined types of rice
- Beans
- Oatmeal
- 100 per cent whole-wheat breads and pasta
- Quinoa
- Barley products (including beer)
- White and sweet potatoes
- Leafy green vegetables

Unprocessed protein

The guidance around protein is much easier to navigate and the advice is clear. Your protein sources should be whole foods (unprocessed) and not contain any additional ingredients. Whole foods that contain protein have a high level of bio availability of that protein, so you really do not need to be supplementing with protein bars and shakes. These products are full of sugar and again provide far less volume per unit of energy than a whole food equivalent. When we think of protein we generally think of meat, but it is important to also note that your sources should contain no extra ingredients, so you should minimise, as tempting as they are, processed meats such as hams, bacon, sausages, salamis and other deli meats. These foods contain numerous chemicals as part of the curing process involved in making them, and the quality and sourcing of the meat used is often debatable, not to mention high in disguised fat.

Your daily protein split should therefore incorporate whole food protein sources such as:

- Lean meats, e.g. beef, pork, lamb
- Poultry, e.g. chicken, turkey and seasonal game birds
- Fish and seafood
- Eggs
- Dairy products
- Tofu
- Tempeh
- Lentils
- Chickpeas and most beans
- Spelt

Good dietary fats

Fat has long been the ugly sister of the primary food groups and swathes of reduced or fat-free products have entered the market to cater to people who want to distance themselves from it. In short, fat is essential to energy balance, and confusion stems from the occurrence of multiple different types of fat. If you ask someone to point to foods high in fat they will probably suggest foods such as pizza, cookies, doughnuts and fried chicken. And they would be right, as all of these foods contain the first of two types of fat, trans fat or trans fatty acids (TFA) to be precise. TFAs are made in an industrial process which involves the hydrogenation (the adding of hydrogen) to vegetable oil to make solid fat for commercial use as a texture and thickening agent in cheap and highly processed foods.[62] In 2013 *TIME* magazine ran a story shining a light on this under-discussed ingredient and found that TFAs are not actually fit for human consumption and should not be in the foods we eat.[63] They campaigned to get the health authorities to make changes, but TFAs in high quantities remain in many foods to this day.

Research has proven a direct correlation between trans fats and cardiovascular disease, breast cancer and the shortening of pregnancy term, not to mention vision development in children, colon cancer and of course weight gain and obesity. It is essential that you avoid trans fats at all costs as the risk-reward is non-existent. Much like smoking, the momentary perceived benefit is immediately outweighed by the immediate onset of dangerous internal mechanisms which risk a reduction in life span. Given this context it is perhaps not so surprising that people err on the side of avoiding fat altogether, but there exists in parallel a branch of fats which are essential for energy balance.

Monounsaturated fat and polyunsaturated fats are also known as unsaturated fats. They are not just a primary source of energy, but they also help the body absorb the fat-soluble vitamins A, D and E and are indispensable for a number of important biological functions such as blood clotting, wound healing and inflammation.

You should therefore ensure that your daily energy split is sourced only from unsaturated fats from food such as:

- Avocados
- Cheese
- >70 per cent cacao dark chocolate
- Eggs (yolk and white)
- Fatty fish, e.g. salmon, mackerel, herring, trout and sardines
- Unsalted and unroasted, shelled nuts
- Chia seeds
- Extra virgin olive oil
- Full-fat yogurt
- Coconuts and coconut oil

It's not the crisps you crave, it's the crunch

Everyone has been guilty of pigging out on a bowl of crisps, popcorn or biscuits in front of a film. Boredom, or eating associated with lazy duvet days off is a principal reason that we gain weight. The mechanism at work here is not actually the treats themselves however, and instead is all about the way they feel in the mouth, or more specifically the crunch. Dr Alan Hirsch explains that humans love crunchy, noisy snacks and what he coins the 'music of mastication'.[64] The research shows that vibrations from the crunch travel down the inner ear to soothe and comfort people and repress feelings of pent-up aggression.

We also associate crunchiness with freshness, and therefore quality, which is a psychology that cereal companies have been cashing in on for years with products which are far from fresh, but draw consumers in with snaps, crackles and pops.

To not miss out on the therapeutic effects of crunchy foods, but not sit on the couch each evening grazing on crisps, opt for equally noisy but healthy snacks such as pickles, rice cakes and whole wheat crackers which you will find equally satisfying.

Marketing campaigns play on our emotions, which can make accurate energy-balancing advice confusing, and government-sponsored campaigns to remedy this in the light of an obesity pandemic are based on advice which is well past its sell-by date. And is counter-intuitive and misguided. Energy balance is very straightforward when you understand the nuances of the primary energy sources: carbohydrates, proteins and fats.

Now that you have your TBMR and clear energy source split you are good to go, right? A number of patients have said that they understand the importance of this, but splitting out the food sources into three equal meals per day seems like hard work, leading many to not try, and to abandon the path to energy balance before it has even begun. We understand that getting three meals exactly right can be challenging to start with, but what if we told you three meals is too many, and that actually two meals a day gets you back to energy balance far quicker and is so much easier to maintain? In the next chapter we will discuss the final element of the energy-balance blueprint by introducing the idea of optimum meal frequency.

9

Optimum Meal Frequency

Many cereal companies will not thank us for saying this, but breakfast is holding you back and making you fat.* A bold claim, but the evidence is resounding that daytime hunger pangs are because you ate breakfast, not the absence of it, and if people struggle to keep their energy intake within their TBMR limit, skipping the toast or cereal will have a huge impact.

Two meals a day

You are going to set yourself an eating window of 7 hours and stick to it. An eating window is the only time frame throughout the day that you have to consume your daily energy intake in line with your TBMR. You can choose any 7-hour slot within the 24 available but we have found most success with those that eat between noon and 7 p.m. This makes the daily energy split far easier to calculate. With a final reference to the 45-year-old woman mentioned throughout, all she needs to do is take her TBMR, which based on Activity Level

---

* It is important that you consult a medical professional before starting any change in your diet, especially if you are diabetic and need to manage blood-sugar levels.

I was 1824kcal energy per day and follow the equation below:

$$1824 \div 2 = 911\text{kcal per meal}$$

Now to work out the energy source split:

$$911 \div 3 = 303.6\text{kcal per energy source}$$

Group	Energy (per gram)
Carbohydrates	4
Fats	9
Proteins	4

So, referring back to the energy source breakdown from Chapter 2, she has to finally divide each energy value by the per energy source total to give her the amount of grams she needs of each to constitute a balanced meal.

Group	Per Meal
Carbohydrates	76g
Fats	33.8g
Proteins	76g

She will only have to do this calculation once every 6 weeks, in line with her updating the TBMR log, and it is a really simple and straightforward framework to ensure energy-balanced meals bespoke to her needs. The strict feeding window means that she (and you) will be fasting for 17 hours every day, which aside from helping you frame your meals much more easily has a host of powerful benefits.

Reduced meal frequency causes your insulin levels to drop, which helps you burn more stored subcutaneous and visceral fat, as well as pushing the body to achieve higher levels of important cell repair processes and remove excess waste from the body. You may think that eating less frequently would go against the common narrative set by body builders and muscle men, that small regular meals are the best way to get lean, and if you are planning to be a professional body builder there is some truth here if the aim is to pack on unhealthy amounts of weight and muscle to your frame. In reality, not eating for over 14 hours each day actually increases human growth hormone in the body five-fold[65] and is a far more effective and balanced approach to gaining lean muscle mass, which not only makes you stronger and more robust, but increases the amount of stored energy you can burn, achieving much needed energy balance far quicker.

The process of reduced meal frequency is known more widely as intermittent fasting and is backed by a growing backlog of supportive evidence and randomised clinical studies. It is also the subject of a number of bestselling diet books including Kate Harrison's *The 5:2 Diet Book* and Dr Michael Mosley and Mimi Spencer's *The Fast Diet*, which have helped millions to reconsider their eating frequency and lose weight.

You might think that the difference between intermittent fasting and reduced meal frequency is down to semantics. And you might be right, however 'fasting' is a very loaded term and one often associated with a start and a finish of say 40 days and 40 nights or a three-month transformation. We believe that this leaves psychological signposting in the mind rather than a wholesale shift in behaviour to eat only within a strict window all the time. And while the diets mentioned, and hosts of others, have impressive short-terms effects, evidenced by numerous success stories, we find that in the months after seeing results the participants often slip back into old habits and in fact gain more weight than they had lost.

Reduced meal frequency to two meals across a maximum of 7 hours is a lifelong commitment, and outside very special and infrequent occasions should be adopted without fail, as slipping back into energy storage is a consequence you cannot afford.

Time to hunt, not time to eat!

We know that the thought of the mid-morning hunger pangs as a result of not eating breakfast might be a little off-putting, but we assure you within three days you won't even think about food until it is time to eat. In fact, people generally find this so easy that they extend their fast to a 4–5-hour eating window as they are simply not hungry until 18 or even 20 hours after their last meal. Importantly though, it is worth mentioning that the feeling of hunger has been very misleadingly defined by the general medical councils of the world, and of course the breakfast cereal companies. Hunger we are told is a signal that we are entering muscle wastage and survival mode that feeds on your hard-fought muscle gains and will leave you limp, exhausted and devoid of energy unless you top yourself up with precious food energy.

You will know from the pages of this book that this is utter nonsense, and while hunger is a signal of survival response, it is not preparing us to eat. Instead, it is the call to arms for us to hunt! In his fantastic book *Lifespan: Why We Age and Why We Don't Have To*, David A. Sinclair PhD says that hunger is not only a good thing, but also triggers a cascade of anti-ageing defences allowing people to turn back the genetic clock as much as 10 years and beyond. He also cites hunger as playing a crucial role in preventing obesity, fighting diabetes, preventing tumour growth and metabolising fat.[66]

The reality is that within three days your body will have recalibrated to the new lifestyle and you won't actually feel hungry at all. But it is still comforting to know that important biological mechanisms are working behind the scenes to reverse the effects of energy storage. Sinclair also argues, which serves as a perfect conclusion to this chapter, that we should all think seriously about 'health span', the amount of time that we have in life fully fit. For decades we have seemingly topped out at a life expectancy of around 90 years old in most best-case scenarios. Yet the litany of injuries, health issues and disease that we endure as a result of gaining and maintaining too much weight means that life after 65 can become a downward spiral resulting in often extremely agonising and exhausting premature death.

Conclusion

At the beginning of this book we made quite clear the world does not need another diet book and we have stayed true to this mantra. We have not pointed to aesthetic cues or get-fit-quick plans for the summer body, and the reasons we hope are perfectly clear. Stopping gaining weight and the reasons you must stop is nothing to do with how you look, the stigma you might be subjected to or the aspirations that the fitness industry convince you are important. Gaining weight is the leading killer of the modern age and makes long, active and fulfilling lives a pipedream. Continuing to gain and maintain excess weight attacks the three core areas of good health – the brain, the cardiovascular system and the lungs – in ways that, if left unchecked, are irreversible and spark the onset of debilitating and all-consuming misery.

Rethinking the problem not as weight gain but of energy storage allows us to better grasp the mechanisms at play. And when we see food not as brightly coloured marketing but as energy derived from three nuanced primary sources – protein, carbohydrates and fats – we can see how easy it actually is to finally implement a strategy that has lifelong staying power.

The blueprint for energy balance shows that with a good plan and a good understanding of why you must act, the process of achieving true energy balance can begin right away. So, with that we thank you for being patrons of this book and we welcome you with open arms to the STOP series community, safe in the knowledge that today is the day you stop gaining weight the easy way.

6-Week Energy Balance Log

As outlined in the book, the things you will need to work out your initial BMR are as follows:

- Body weight scales (analogue or digital)
- Measuring tape
- Calculator
- Pen/pencil

Please take and record the following data points:

Weight (kg)		Height (cm)		Age (years)	

Now apply the following formula to the data points above

A	**10** × your body **weight** in kilograms =	
B	**6.25** × your **height** in centimetres =	
C	**5** × your **age** =	

Next, put your A, B and C totals into the following equation to get your specific BMR and note that there is a slight difference in equation for men and women.

Women: A + B − C − 161 = BMR
Men: A + B − C + 51 = BMR

Day one BMR:

Finally, reference the activity-level scale below and multiply your BMR by the factor which most accurately describes your daily life, and please be honest!

Activity Level	Description	TBMR
1 Little to non-existent	No exercise at all	TBMR = BMR × 1.2
2 Light (average)	Walking 1–3 times a week	TBMR = BMR × 1.375
3 Moderate	Sports or gym >3 a week	TBMR = BMR × 1.55
4 High	High intensity >5 a week	TBMR = BMR × 1.75
5 Extreme	Training twice a day	TBMR = BMR × 1.9

Day one TBMR:

Excellent, you have now calculated your day 1 TBMR. This is the critical first step in the journey towards true energy balance.

Now enter the information in the first cell of the 6-Week Energy Balance Log below, and continue to make this calculation in 6 week intervals to monitor how your TBMR changes over time. Remember you must always be honest about your true activity level at all times.

Week	Date	BMR	Activity level	TBMR
6				
12				
18				
24				
30				
36				

Walking Tracker

As we discussed in Part 2, recording daily walks helps those less used to regular exercise to move up through the activity levels and reap the huge health benefits it brings. For any reader who on day one is defined by either Activity Level 1 or 2, please follow the walking routine outlined below, checking the box in the 'completed' column each day. Please do keep a record of your thoughts on progress in the notes, and should you miss a day (which we know you won't) please record the reasons why.

Week 1

DAY	TARGET (minutes)	COMPLETED (Y/N)	NOTES
1	11		
2	11		
3	11		
4	11		
5	11		
6	11		
7	11		

Week 2

DAY	TARGET (minutes)	COMPLETED (Y/N)	NOTES
8	11		
9	11		
10	11		
11	11		
12	11		
13	11		
14	11		

Week 3

DAY	TARGET (minutes)	COMPLETED (Y/N)	NOTES
15	20		
16	20		
17	20		
18	20		
19	20		
20	30		
21	Rest day		

Week 4

DAY	TARGET (minutes)	COMPLETED (Y/N)	NOTES
22	20		
23	20		
24	20		
25	20		
26	20		
27	30		
28	Rest day		

Congratulations! You have just completed the 4 weeks of Walking Activity 1. In this time, you will have walked for a minimum of 17 hours and we hope taken great benefit from time outdoors, away from screens and in the fresh air. Your progress means you are now ready for Activity Level 2. Please remember to recalculate your TBMR and record it in the 6-Week Energy Balance Log.

What follows is the base level activity to maintain Activity Level 2, so ensure you keep up the week 5 routine as a bare minimum.

Week 5

DAY	TARGET (minutes)	COMPLETED (Y/N)	NOTES	
29	35			
30	35			
31	35			
32	35			
33	35			
34	60			
35	Rest day			

If you'd like to continue beyond Week 5, then use this blank table as a template for further weeks to track your progress.

DAY	TARGET (minutes)	COMPLETED (Y/N)	NOTES					

References

1 https://fdocuments.net/document/colon-hydrotherapy-is-a-scientificaly-essene-gospel-of-peace-book-one-by-edmond.html?page=1

2 https://www.who.int/news-room/fact-sheets/detail/obesity-and-overweight

3 https://dentistry.co.uk/2020/05/05/latest-nhs-figures-children-obese/

4 https://www.gov.uk/government/publications/health-matters-obesity-and-the-food-environment

5 www.healthline.com/health-news/worried-about-weight-gain-during-covid-19-physicians-say-youre-not-alone

6 ibid.

7 Galgani J., Ravussin E., 'Energy metabolism, fuel selection and body weight regulation'. Int J Obes (Lond). 2008 Dec;32 Suppl 7(Suppl 7):S109-S119. doi:10.1038/ijo.2008.246

8 https://www.healthline.com/nutrition/calorie-restriction-risks#TOC_TITLE_HDR_6

9 https://theconversation.com/stored-fat-is-a-feat-of-evolution-and-your-body-will-fight-to-keep-it-52468

10 Ludwig D.S., Hu F.B., Tappy L., Brand-Miller J. 'Dietary carbohydrates: role of quality and quantity in chronic disease', BMJ. 2018;361:k2340. Published 2018 Jun 13. doi:10.1136/bmj.k2340

11 ibid

12 https://www.hsph.harvard.edu/nutritionsource/carbohydrates/carbohydrates-and-blood-sugar/

13 Chianese R., Coccurello R., Viggiano A., et al. 'Impact of Dietary Fats on Brain Functions'. Curr Neuropharmacol. 2018;16(7):1059-1085. doi:10.2174/1570159X15666171017102547

14 Carbone J.W., Pasiakos S.M. 'Dietary Protein and Muscle Mass: Translating Science to Application and Health Benefit'. Nutrients. 2019;11(5):1136. Published 2019 May 22. doi:10.3390/nu11051136

15 ibid.

16 https://inbodyusa.com/blogs/inbodyblog/49311425-how-to-use-bmr-to-hack-your-diet/

17 https://thewellnessconnection.com/optimal-health-manifesto/#:~:text=A%20
state%20of%20complete%20well,absence%20of%20disease%20or%20
infirmity.

18 Lodish H., Berk A., Zipursky S.L., et al. Molecular Cell Biology. 4th edition. New
York: W. H. Freeman; 2000. Section 21.1, 'Overview of Neuron Structure and
Function'. Available from: https://www.ncbi.nlm.nih.gov/books/NBK21535/

19 Gorelick P.B., Furie K.L., Iadecola C., et al. 'Defining Optimal Brain Health
in Adults: A Presidential Advisory From the American Heart Association/
American Stroke Association'. Stroke. 2017;48(10):e284-e303. doi:10.1161/
STR.0000000000000148

20 https://www.livescience.com/39925-circulatory-system-facts-surprising.html

21 https://curesearch.org/Blood-Studies

22 https://www.osmosis.org/answers/lividity

23 https://www.britannica.com/science/human-cardiovascular-system

24 http://www.upbeatheartsupport.org.uk/theheartfactsfigures.html

25 https://doi.org/10.1152/advances.2000.24.1.43

26 Delgado B.J., Bajaj T. 'Physiology, Lung Capacity'. [Updated 2020 Aug 11]. In:
StatPearls [Internet]. Treasure Island (FL): StatPearls Publishing; 2021 Jan-.
Available from: https://www.ncbi.nlm.nih.gov/books/NBK541029/

27 https://www.medicalnewstoday.com/articles/305190#surfactant

28 https://www.sciencedaily.com/releases/2020/08/200805110127.htm#:~:
text=Summary%3A,a%20new%20brain%20imaging%20study.&text=FULL
%20STORY-As%20a%20person's%20weight%20goes%20up%2C%20all%20
regions%20of%20the,the%20Journal%20of%20Alzheimer's%20Disease.

29 https://practicalneurology.com/articles/2013-july-aug/the-effects-of-obesity-
on-brain-structure-and-size

30 https://newsroom.saga.co.uk/news/dementia-more-feared-than-cancer-new-
saga-survey-reveals

31 https://www.ucl.ac.uk/news/2020/jun/obesity-linked-higher-dementia-risk

32 https://www.niddk.nih.gov/health-information/health-statistics/overweight-
obesity

33 Mittal B., 'Subcutaneous adipose tissue & visceral adipose tissue'. Indian J Med
Res. 2019;149(5):571-573. doi:10.4103/ijmr.IJMR_1910_18

34 https://www.diabetes.co.uk/insulin-resistance.html

35 https://medschool.vanderbilt.edu/vanderbilt-medicine/the-good-the-bad-and-the-ugly-of-inflammation/#:~:text=When%20it's%20good%2C%20it%20fights,possibly%2C%20autism%20and%20mental%20illness.

36 Coryell W.H., Butcher B.D., Burns T.L., Dindo L.N., Schlechte J.A., Calarge C.A., 'Fat distribution and major depressive disorder in late adolescence'. J Clin Psychiatry. 2016;77(1):84-89. doi:10.4088/JCP.14m09169

37 https://www.health.harvard.edu/staying-healthy/abdominal-fat-and-what-to-do-about-it

38 https://www.bhf.org.uk/what-we-do/news-from-the-bhf/contact-the-press-office/facts-and-figures

39 ibid.

40 Dixon A.E., Peters U., 'The effect of obesity on lung function'. Expert Rev Respir Med. 2018;12(9):755-767. doi:10.1080/17476348.2018.1506331

41 Mafort T.T., Rufino R., Costa C.H. et al., 'Obesity: systemic and pulmonary complications, biochemical abnormalities, and impairment of lung function'. Multidiscip Respir Med 11, 28 (2016). https://doi.org/10.1186/s40248-016-0066-z

42 Peralta G.P., Marcon A., Carsin A., et al., 'Body mass index and weight change are associated with adult lung function trajectories: the prospective ECRHS study'. Thorax 2020;75:313-320.

43 van der Gugten A.C., Koopman M., Evelein A.M., Verheij T.J., Uiterwaal C.S., van der Ent C.K., 'Rapid early weight gain is associated with wheeze and reduced lung function in childhood'. Eur Respir J. 2012 Feb;39(2):403-10. doi: 10.1183/09031936.00188310. Epub 2011 Aug 18. PMID: 21852338.

44 https://www.mirror.co.uk/tv/tv-news/jesy-nelson-attempted-suicide-after-19972725

45 https://yougov.co.uk/topics/lifestyle/articles-reports/2020/01/23/nearly-half-brits-are-unhappy-their-body

46 https://theconversation.com/half-of-employers-say-they-are-less-inclined-to-recruit-obese-candidates-its-not-ok-109821

47 https://asdah.org/how-we-can-reframe-gaining-weight-as-an-act-of-self-care/

48 https://www.reuters.com/article/uk-factcheck-94-percent-covid-among-caus-idUSKBN25U2I0

49 Basen-Engquist K., Chang M., 'Obesity and cancer risk: recent review and evidence'. Curr Oncol Rep. 2011;13(1):71-76. doi:10.1007/s11912-010-0139-7

50 https://www.cancer.gov/about-cancer/causes-prevention/risk/obesity/obesity-fact-sheet

51 https://www.cdc.gov/vitalsigns/obesity-cancer/infographic.html#graphic

52 ibid.

53 https://www.hsph.harvard.edu/news/hsph-in-the-news/binge-watching-tv-not-good-for-waistline/

54 Neovius M., Sundström J., Rasmussen F., 'Combined effects of overweight and smoking in late adolescence on subsequent mortality: nationwide cohort study'. BMJ 2009; 338 :b496 doi:10.1136/bmj.b496

55 https://www.drinkaware.co.uk/research/research-and-evaluation-reports/alcohol-consumption-uk

56 https://www.nuffieldtrust.org.uk/resource/alcohol-related-harm-and-drinking-behaviour-1#:~:text=In%20England%2C%20the%20alcohol%2Drelated,%25%2C%20but%20fluctuated%20over%20time.

57 van der Valk E.S., Savas M., van Rossum E.F.C., 'Stress and Obesity: Are There More Susceptible Individuals?'. Curr Obes Rep. 2018;7(2):193-203. doi:10.1007/s13679-018-0306-y

58 https://www.healthline.com/nutrition/cortisol-and-weight-gain#effects-on-weight

59 https://www.therecoveryvillage.com/mental-health/stress/related/stress-statistics/#:~:text=According%20to%20The%20American%20Institute,that%20impacts%20their%20mental%20health

60 https://www.health.harvard.edu/blog/10000-steps-a-day-or-fewer-2019071117305

61 https://www.nutrition.org.uk/healthyliving/healthydiet.html?gclid=Cj0KCQjwl9GCBhDvARIsAFunhsl-71bFW42syJQ-3HBzGgtgZW3UBFNyoizXYB2XOAdJgycBWsjQh64aAruVEALw_wcB

62 Dhaka V., Gulia N., Ahlawat K.S., Khatkar B.S., 'Trans fats – sources, health risks and alternative approach – A review'. J Food Sci Technol. 2011;48(5):534-541. doi:10.1007/s13197-010-0225-8

63 https://healthland.time.com/2013/11/07/7-foods-that-wont-be-the-same-if-trans-fats-are-banned/

64 https://www.mentalfloss.com/article/531186/science-behind-why-we-crave-loud-and-crunchy-foods

65 https://www.healthline.com/nutrition/10-health-benefits-of-intermittent-fasting#TOC_TITLE_HDR_2

66 https://hms.harvard.edu/magazine/food-issue/stone-soup

STOP
GAINING WEIGHT